I0417649

TAPE 'N CUT

Do It Yourself Hair – Instruction Booklet

*An Inexpensive, Fast and Safe
Way to Cut Hair*

Sabrina R. Denebeim

1st Edition

© Copyright 1999-2017 Sabrina R. Denebeim
All Rights Reserved

No part of this publication may be reproduced, stored in a retrieval system, or trans-mitted in any form or by any means, electronic, mechanical, recording or otherwise without prior written permission of the author.

Also available as an ebook

TAPE 'N CUT

TABLE OF CONTENTS

INTRODUCTION

TAPE 'N CUT is an inexpensive, fast and safe way to cut hair. **TAPE 'N CUT** can be adapted to various hair lengths and textures.

TAPE 'N CUT achieves high quality, stylish results. You can easily cut hair by attaching tape to the hair above the length you want, then immediately follow **TAPE 'N CUT's** instructions and illustrations as a guide.

All you need to cut hair is:
- Scissors
- Comb
- Masking tape or hair tape

Tip:
You can purchase hair setting tape in the hair accessory aisle at most drug stores.

IMPORTANT
SAFETY INSTRUCTIONS

(Read **before** cutting)

General Haircutting Tips

1. Hair can be cut wet or dry.

2. Cut the bangs first.

3. The tape should be cut longer than the area cut. Two pieces of tape together are more secure. If the tape is not secure, attach the tape (or new tape) again.

4. Cut from one side across to the other.

5. When cutting around the ears, be extra careful. The tape can help hold the ears in place.

6. Do not put too much hair into one cut of the scissors.

7. Hair does not vacuum well. Sweep or place something on the floor.

8. Highchairs are ideal for toddlers.

9. If the child becomes restless, stop cutting. You can finish at another time.

10. Scissors are sharp.

11. Avoid eye area.

BANGS
Blunt-Cut Bangs

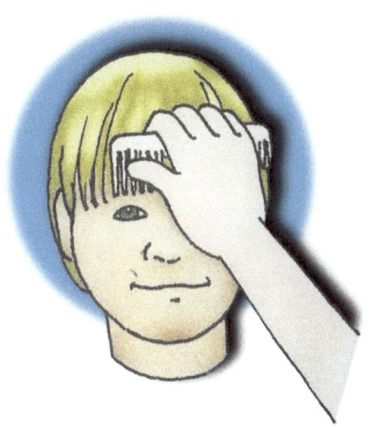 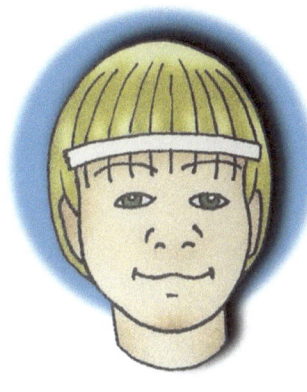

Blunt-Cut Bangs

1. Comb the bangs over the forehead.

2. Attach the tape slightly above the eyebrows, starting from one side of the head and extending to the other side.

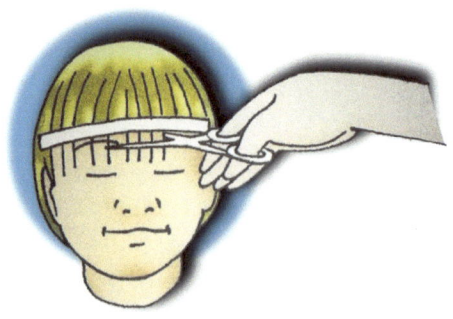 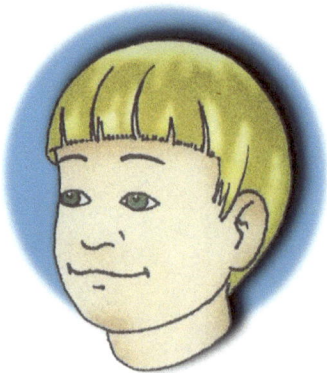

3. Cut across the bangs, underneath the tape, starting at the eyebrows.

4. Remove the tape.

Tip:
Leave the bangs longer if there is a heavy front cowlick.

BANGS
WISPY BANGS

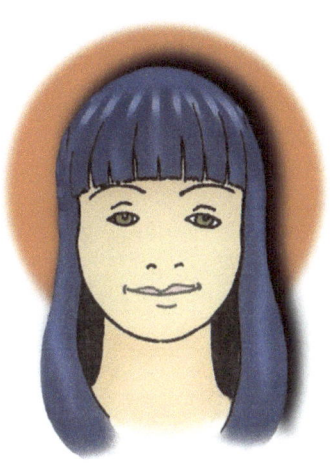 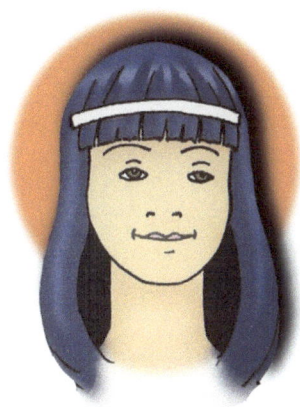

Wispy Bangs

1. Comb the bangs over the forehead.

2. Attach the tape slightly above the eyebrows, starting from one side of the head and extending to the other side.

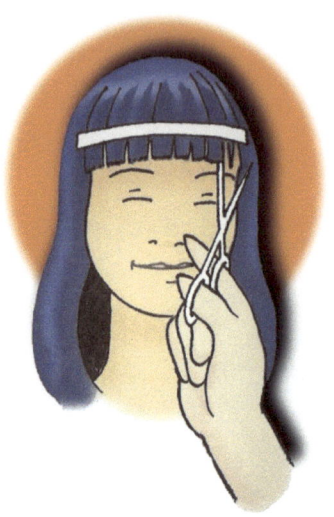 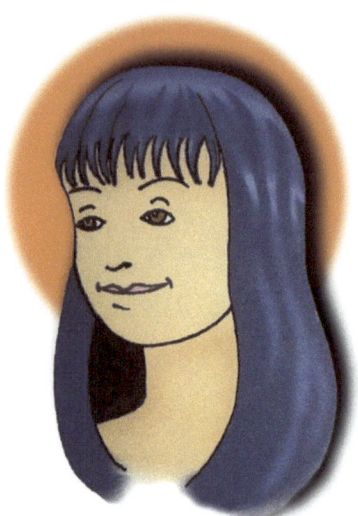

3. Cut straight up, into the bangs, **underneath** the tape. Repeat the straight up cut across the bangs. The wispy bangs have a sawtooth or VVV shape. The wispier the cut, the more VVVs are required.

4. Remove the tape.

Tip:
Leave the bangs longer if there is a heavy front cowlick.

HAIRCUT
ONE-LENGTH CUT

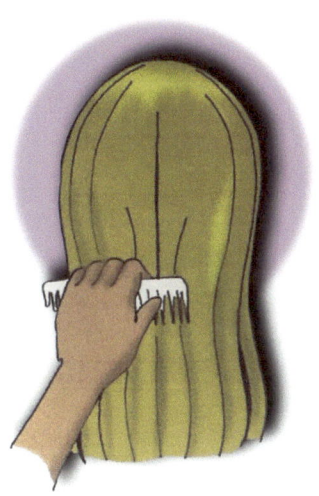
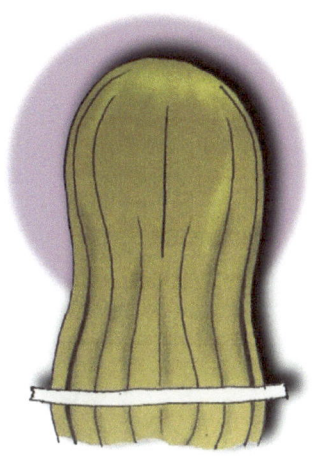

One-Length Cut (shoulders and below) (with or without blunt or wispy bangs)

1. Cut the bangs first if desired.

2. Comb all the hair straight down so it falls over the shoulders and across the back.

3. Attach a long piece of tape from one shoulder to the other, slightly **above** the desired length.

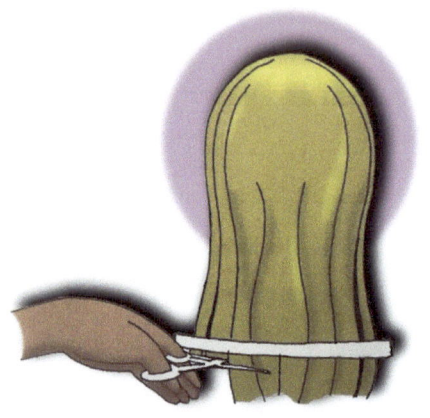 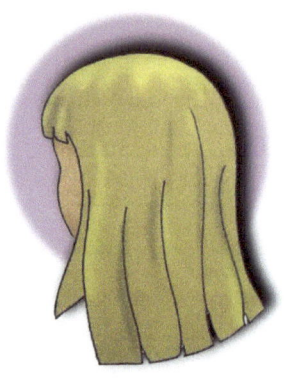

4. Cut from one side, underneath the tape, across to the other side.

5. Remove the tape.

HAIRCUT
Long or Short Bob

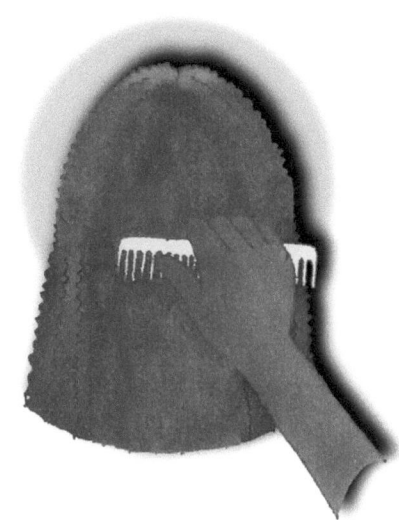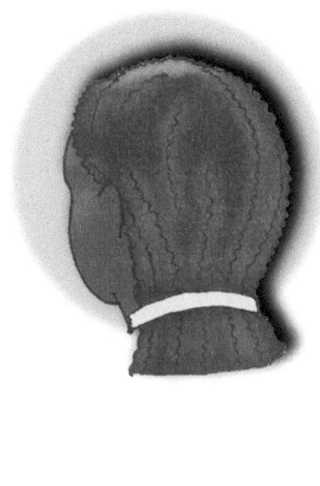

Short Bob (above the shoulders) (with or without blunt or wispy bangs) or right above the shoulders for a longer bob.

1. Cut the bangs first, if desired.

2. Comb all the hair straight down.

3. Attach the tape around each side of the neck to form a collar.

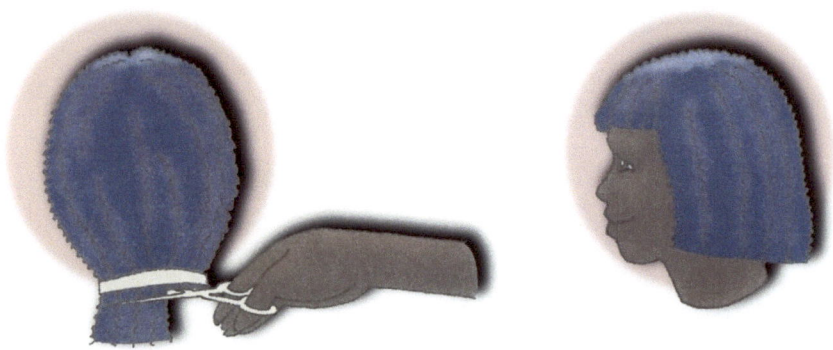

4. Cut from one side, underneath the tape, across to the other side.

5. Remove the tape.

Tip:
Attach the tape around the back of the head, from chin to chin or cheek to cheek for a shorter haircut.

HAIRCUT
Bowl Cut
GIRL OR BOY

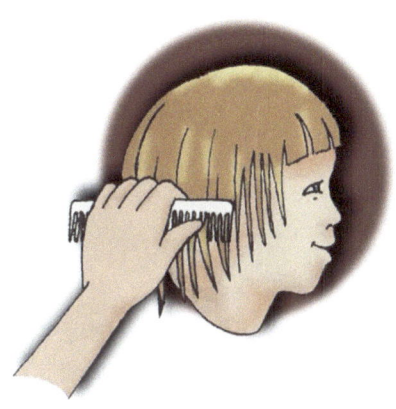
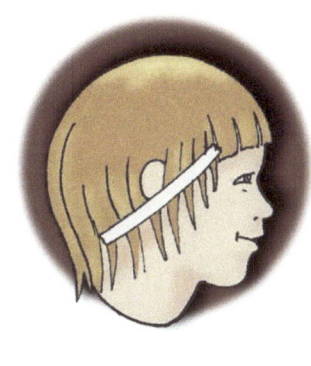

Bowl (Bangs are required.)

1. Cut the bangs first.

2. Comb the hair downward on one side.

3. Angle the **first** tape downward, from the end of the bangs, across or above the ear, to the back of the neck.

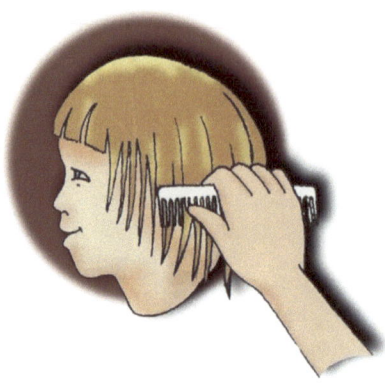 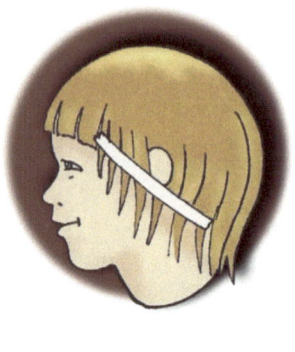

4. Comb the hair downward on the other side

5. Angle the second tape downward, from the end of the bangs, across or above the ear, to the back of the neck.

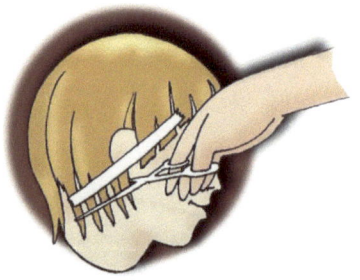 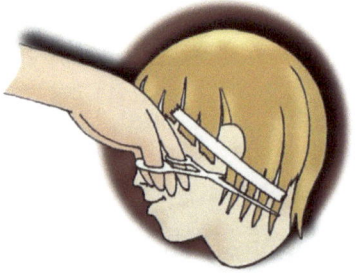

6. Cut underneath the first tape.

7. Cut underneath the second tape.

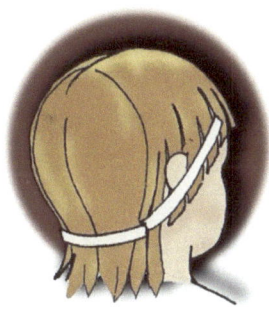 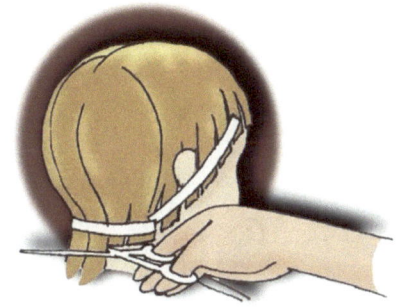

8. Attach the third tape across the back of the neck (or shoulders).

9. Cut **underneath** the **third** tape, straight across.

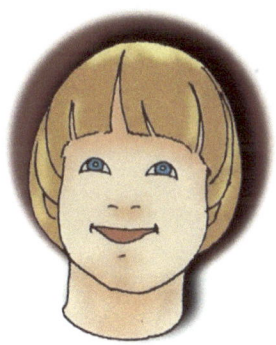

10. Remove all **three** tapes.

Tip:
Cut the neck hairs if desired.

HAIRCUT
Short Wedge Cut
GIRL OR BOY

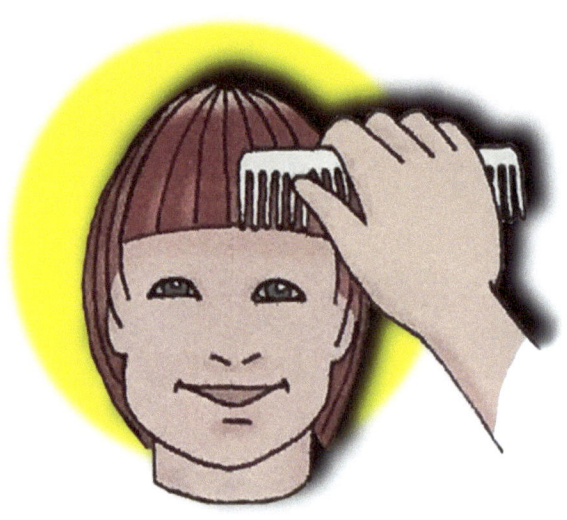

Short Cut (Bangs are required.)

1. Cut the bangs first.

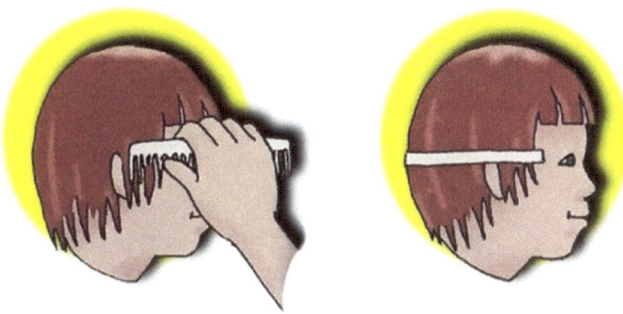

2. Comb the hair downward on one side.

3. Attach the **first** tape from the ends of the bangs (or cheekbone) to the middle of the back of the head.

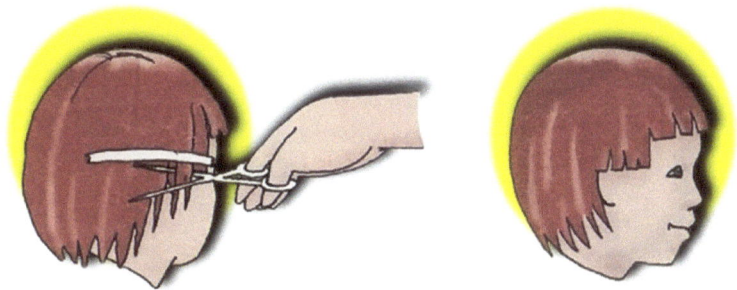

4. Cut straight across, **underneath** the **first** tape, from the ends of the bangs, (or cheekbone) **above** the ear, ending just behind the ear. Do **not** cut to the middle of the back!

5. Remove the **first** tape.

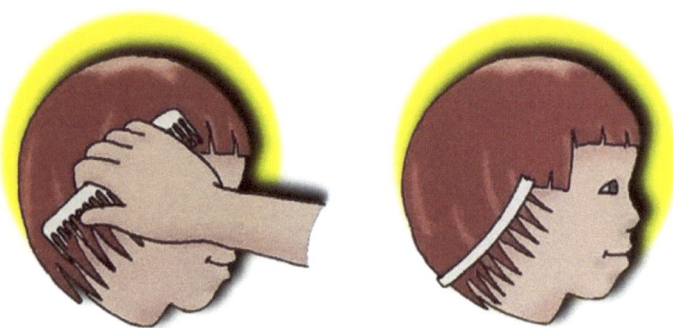

6. Comb the hair that remains behind the ear towards the face.

7. Angle the **second** tape downward, from above the ear, to the middle of the back of the head.

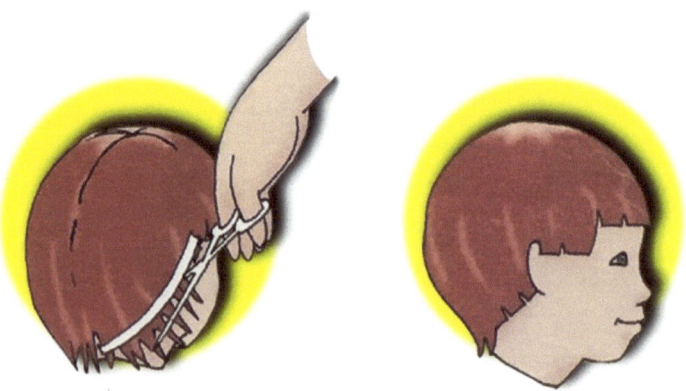

8. Cut **downward**, underneath the **second** tape.

9. Remove the **second** tape.

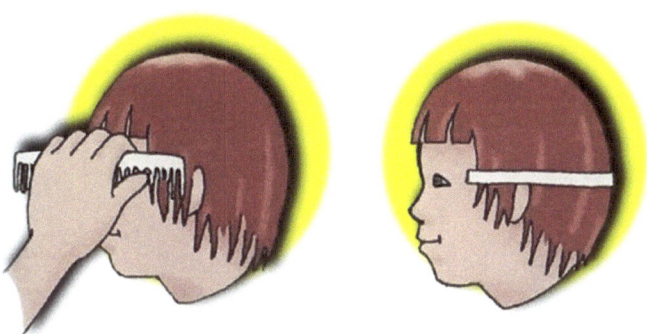

10. Comb the hair downward on the **other side**.

11. From the **other side**, attach the **third** tape from the ends of the bangs (or cheekbone) to the middle of the back of the head.

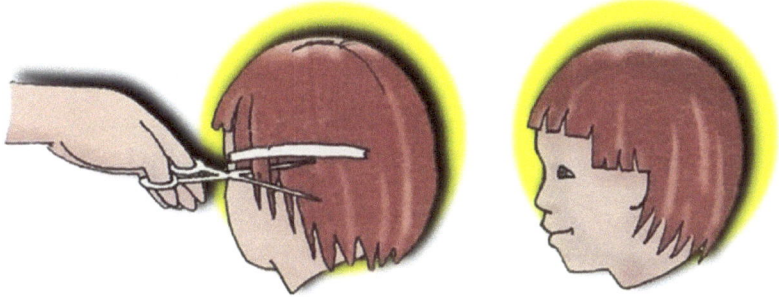

12. Cut straight across, **underneath** the **third** tape, from the ends of the bangs, (or cheekbone) **above** the ear, ending just behind the ear. Do **not** cut to the middle of the back!

13. Remove the **third** tape.

19

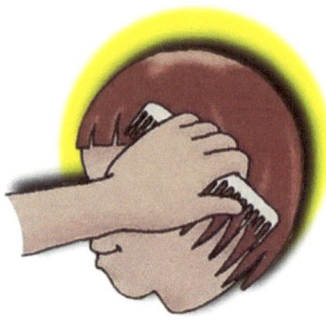
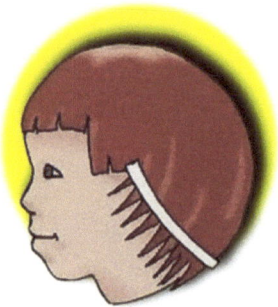

14. Comb the hair on the **other side** that remains behind the ear towards the face.

15. Angle the **fourth** tape downward, from above the ear, to the middle of the back of the head.

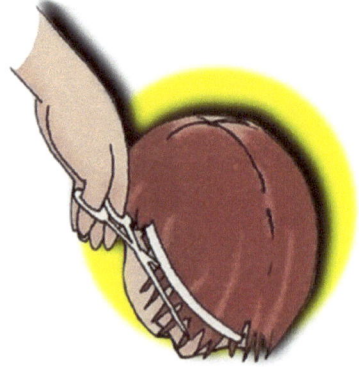
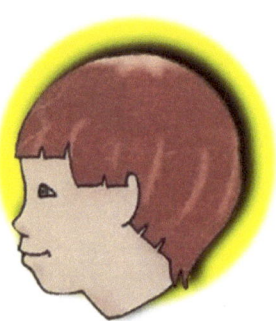

16. Cut **downward**, underneath the **fourth** tape.

17. Remove the **fourth** tape.

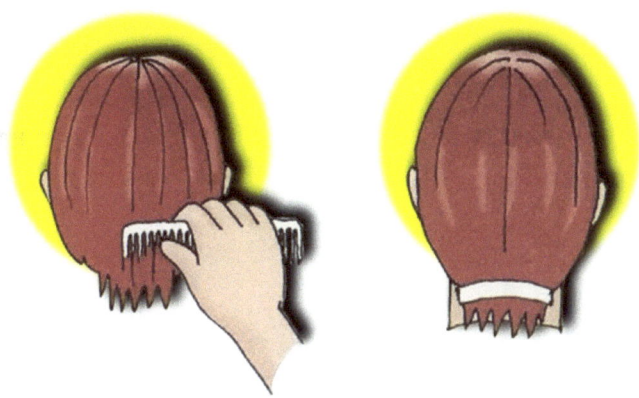

18. Comb the hair in the back downward.

19. Attach the **fifth** tape across the back of the neck.

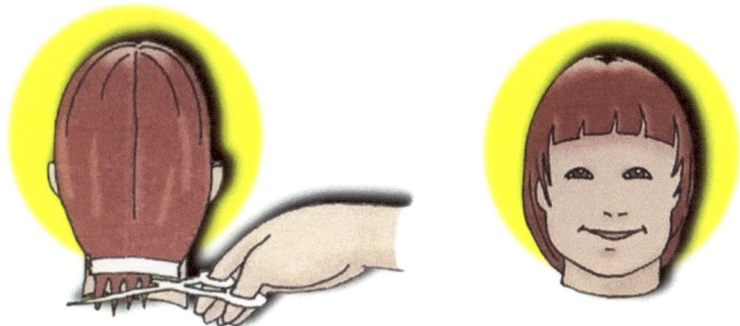

20. Cut from one side, **underneath** the **fifth** tape, to the other side.

21. Remove the **fifth** tape.

Tip:
Attach the fifth tape higher for a shorter back, or lower for a longer back.

ABOUT THE AUTHOR

An esteemed Hairstylist and Inventor, **Sabrina Denebeim** has worked with many celebrities, including athletes, actors, and politicians. While enjoying her profession, she developed her passion for designing hair products and was awarded her first patent in 1990. Since then, she has accumulated over 16 more patents in the years that followed. Her patented inventions embody a wide range of designs, including many styles of hairbrushes, rollers and other hair accessories and tools.

Sabrina has designed and licensed products for Scunci, Helen of Troy, Conair and won the Bed Bath & Beyond *Product of the Year* award. She has developed product lines for well-known celebrities such as Paris Hilton and Jessica Simpson. Her products have been featured on QVC and various major magazines, including Vogue, Women's Home Journal, WWD, and many others. Her products have appeared in movies and even been mocked on David Letterman.

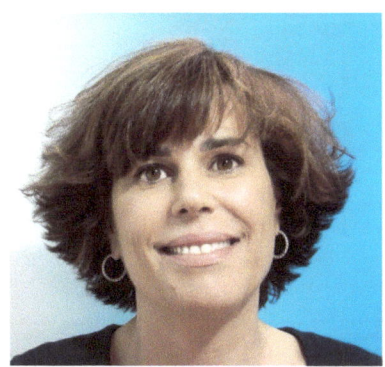

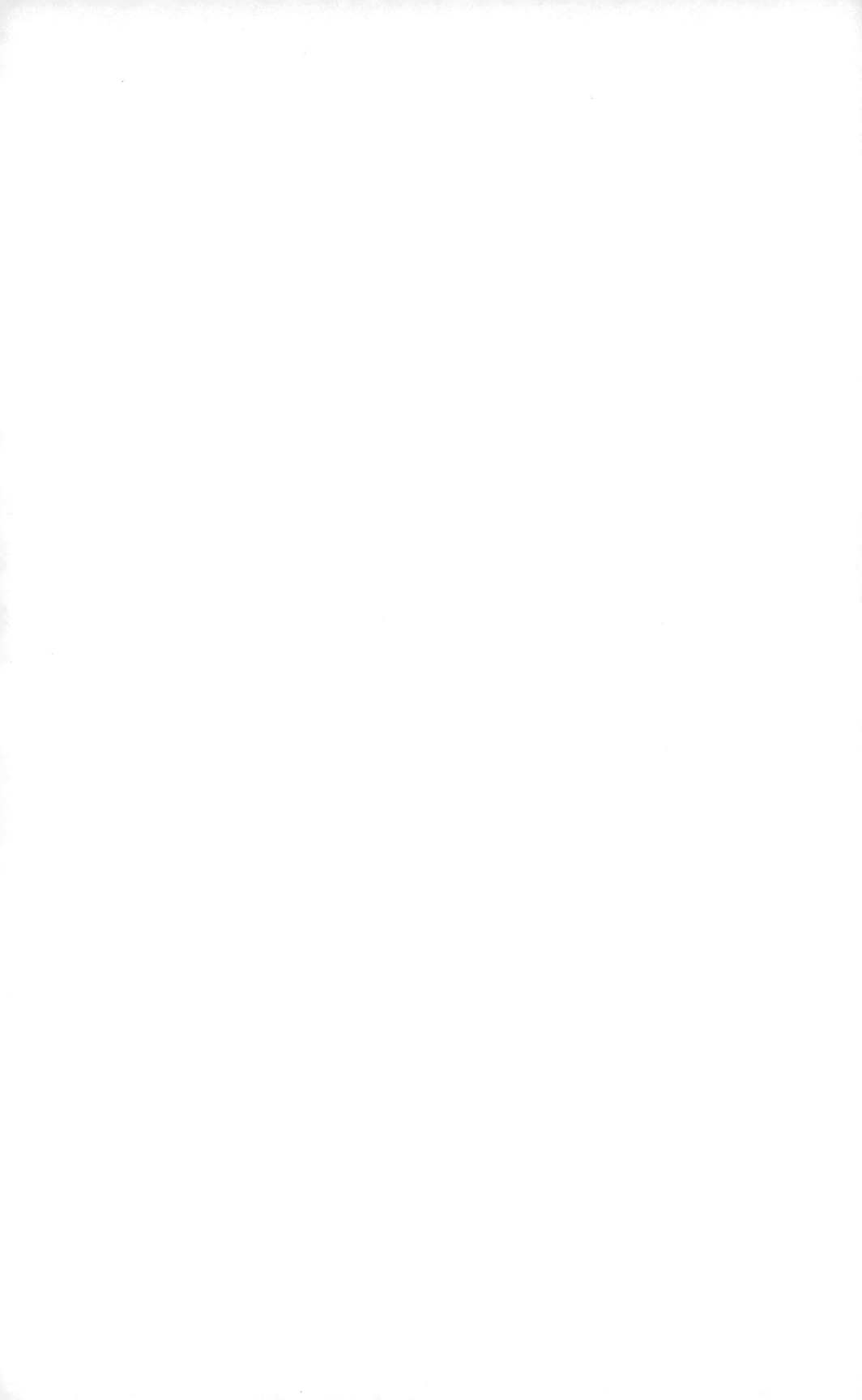

www.ingramcontent.com/pod-product-compliance
Lightning Source LLC
Chambersburg PA
CBHW050928290526
45792CB00002B/930